1.75

ABOUT DEVIL'S CLAW

Tells the story of this strange African plant, which protects its seed with a vicious claw, and which yields from its tubers a substance which offers relief to sufferers from rheumatic and arthritic conditions.

By the same author
ABOUT THE SALT OF LIFE
THE CIDER VINEGAR AND MOLASSES
RECIPE BOOK
HANSSEN'S COMPLETE CIDER VINEGAR
THE BLENDER AND JUICER BOOK

Co-authored with Jack Eden
NATURAL COLD CURES

Co-authored with Jacqueline Dineen
WINES, BEERS AND SPIRITS

ABOUT DEVIL'S CLAW

The Natural and Safe Treatment of Rheumatism and Arthritis

by
MAURICE HANSSEN

THORSONS PUBLISHERS LIMITED
Wellingborough, Northamptonshire

First published 1978

ISBN 0 7225 0450 0

Photoset by
Specialised Offset Services Ltd, Liverpool
Printed and bound in Great Britain by
Weatherby Woolnough, Wellingborough,
Northamptonshire

CONTENTS

ACKNOWLEDGEMENT

The author thanks Herr Otto Greither and his colleagues at Salus-Haus in Bruckmühl, West Germany, for the considerable help they gave him in the difficult task of tracking down the many medical and pharmacological references used in the writing of this book.

INTRODUCTION

I have written this book because a close study of all the available medical and pharmaceutical papers written between 1958 and 1977 on the subject has convinced me that Devil's Claw (*Harpagophytum procumbens*) is a very important and safe herb for the treatment of rheumatism and arthritis.

A famous London teaching hospital is currently carrying out trials, repeating and extending on from those already made in Germany, and first indications are promising – although research is not likely to be concluded for several years. In the meantime, however, there is a need for sufferers from rheumatic and arthritic conditions to be made aware of the developments so far in the understanding of this new therapy.

Until now information has largely been spread by word of mouth and, apart from an informative leaflet by Hildegard Pickles, nothing has been published for popular readership. British medical regulations prevent importers and processors of Devil's Claw from making any claims at all as to the effectiveness of the plant, and they are not likely to be able to do so at least until the London trials have been concluded.

It is, therefore, my hope that the information in this book will enable many more than at present to take advantage of Devil's Claw, and I also hope that it will bring to the attention of Medical Research Units everywhere the need to investigate this plant.

Sadly, as with almost any treatment, some will find no help or relief. For them researchers will continue to seek answers. But to those who try Devil's Claw and benefit I dedicate this book. Be aware, though, that to be fully effective the product must be derived from the secondary roots or tubers of the plant. The main or primary root contains at best one half of the active substances found in the secondary root, so I urge you to read the packet carefully before you buy and ensure that the product you use is prepared exclusively from the secondary roots or tubers, or else you may be needlessly disappointed with the results.

CHAPTER ONE

THE ORIGIN OF DEVIL'S CLAW

Africa is not a hospitable land. There is natural beauty in abundance, but dangers seen and unseen forever threaten the security of those who live in or venture to the dark continent; not just disease, pestilence and plague, but the ferocity of animal and insect life. Lethally poisonous snakes lay coiled and comatose, and scorpions scurry about their business, but should you stumble unwittingly into their domain they will strike violently and fatally since their venom is so toxic that when stung your very minutes become numbered.

It is little wonder that those who survive in this hostile environment are observant to a degree unknown in the Western World. A sixth sense built up over endless generations of experience enables life to go on; and indeed to flourish.

Such sharpened awareness has not been concerned only with animal and insect life, and there has also developed over the ages a rapport with and respect for the plants and trees that grow lustily and in a profusion of colour and variety in these tropical regions: from the tangled and near-impenetrable jungle to the sparse vegetation of the low-rainfall scrublands and deserts.

In the same way as all other forms of life that have battled for a right to survive in this land of extremes, the plants have developed their own highly sophisticated defence and propagation mechanisms, and man's knowledge of them has been built up mainly by the results of direct experience – an increasing fund of wisdom being passed from generation to generation by word of mouth.

Perhaps ten thousand years ago, or even a hundred thousand, a dark-skinned hunting male of the human species, with crude spear held at his shoulder, increased his pace as he broke cover and headed speedily and intently across the scrub at the edge of what is now known as the Kalahari desert in pursuit of his fleet-footed prey – a prey he had been stalking for hours, and which had drawn the huntsman further from his home ground than he had ever strayed before.

He was now running, and his feet struck the sandy soil heavily and rhythmically as he closed for the kill. Suddenly he stumbled and fell; his spear flying from his grasp as he slithered and rolled to a stop, showering sand ahead of him and sending his prey cantering off to safety. He was hurt; pain was shooting up his right leg. He clasped his foot which seemed to be gripped in vice-like jaws.

He pulled his injured foot towards him, and to his surprise found that imbedded in his flesh was a strange barbed claw belonging to an attractive plant with purple trumpet-shaped flowers and small leaves on trailing green stems. He had never seen such a plant before – unwittingly he had invaded its privacy and had paid the price.

That night the huntsman hobbled home

without fresh meat, but perhaps with something far more valuable. He had discovered *Harpagophytum procumbens* – more descriptively known as Devil's Claw; a name which cannot be far from that given to it by its primitive discoverer. That hunter and his kin would respect this strange toothed plant from now on.

Vicious Talons

As I write, there are before me two dried Devil's Claws from the Namibian Plains of South West Africa. They look like long-dead spiders with sixteen legs instead of eight. One is five inches (13cm) across, and the other about half that size. The 'legs' curve upward from the ground to form a bowl, and each leg bears, at intervals, dreadful and deeply downward curving thorns like vicious talons.

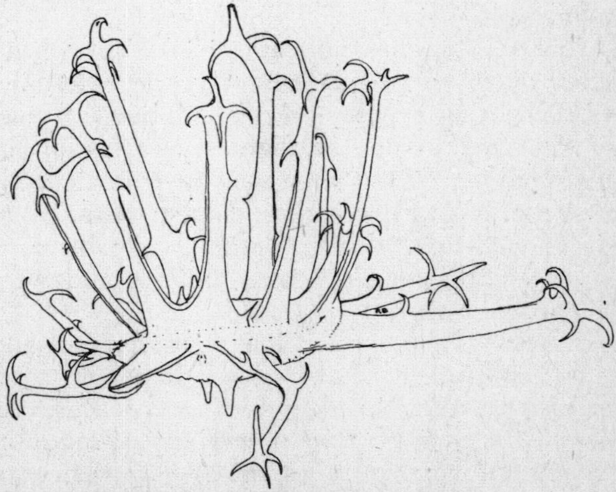

The barbed claw of the Devil's Claw plant.

However delicately I move these claws, the angles at which the barbs are set inevitably mean that they have to be unhooked from my skin as they are put down again. The dark-green living claws are not only just as brutally sharp as my dried specimens but, when trodden on, all the arms curve in and penetrate the foot so strongly that today iron tools are employed to release the injured part. Our lone huntsman of long ago will have spent hours painfully removing the Devil's Claw from his heel before limping back to warn the other members of his tribe of this new danger.

Sympathetic Magic

Was it then perhaps sympathetic magic that eventually led some witch doctor to seek a cure for sufferers from rheumatic and arthritic joints in just that plant that could cause such havoc and pain to the foot?

The idea that plants with medical powers do often show these qualities in some externally visible feature is of the greatest antiquity. It may be that there is not the slightest justification for the relationhsip, but what may have happened is that plants with interesting characteristics were tried out first. Some worked, and became accepted treatments, others did not and were discarded.

Bryony root is shaped like a swollen foot and was considered good for dropsy (water retention), and as *Potter's New Cyclopaedia of Botanical Drugs and Preparations* also points out, plants with yellow flowers, roots or sap were used for jaundice; red roots for bleeding, and poplar leaves – called Quaking Aspen because of the strange way in which they shake in the breeze – for palsy.

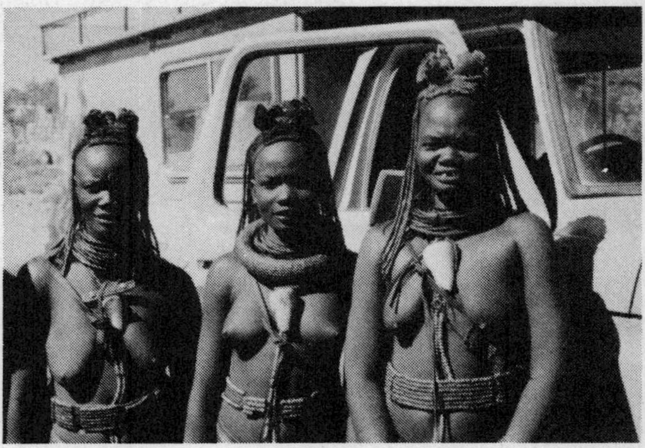

These Ovahimba girls are typical of the strong and healthy people from the areas where Devil's Claw flourishes. Along with the women of the Namas in the south, and Herreros and Ovambos to the north of Namibia, the Ovahimbos find that the herb relieves the pains of pregnancy.

Certainly, the root of Devil's Claw became a folk remedy with an anti-rheumatic effect amongst the native Africans of Namibia, and it has been used by them for generations. Time will perhaps show how many of the other African uses of this plant will be recognized and adopted by European medicine – such uses as a treatment for indigestion, blood diseases, fever, pain and certain complications of pregnancy. The fresh tuber is also made into an ointment for treating skin complaints, and yet other claims include its use as a remedy for poor assimilation of food, as a treatment (under medical control) for diabetes, for liver, gall, nerves and lung problems, for gout, allergies and premature ageing. A formidable list, indeed, and it will take researchers very many years to learn in which of these conditions *Harpagophytum procumbens* is really effective. The safety factor of the tuber (no side-effects) as against synthesized drugs is surely an encouragement to research.

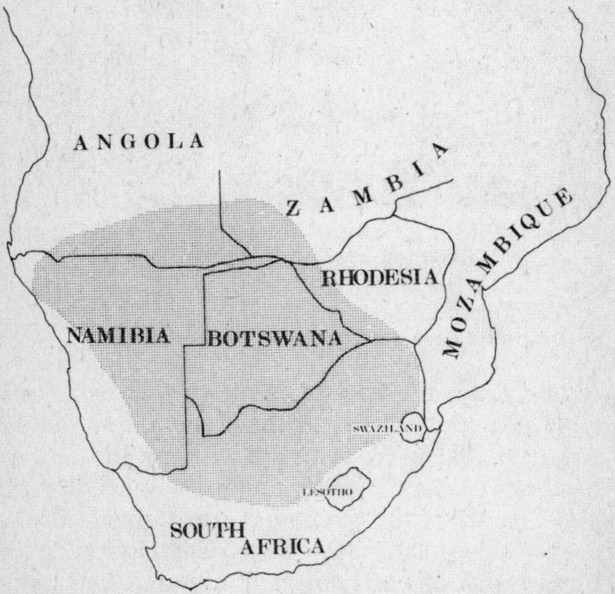

Map showing the areas in which Devil's Claw grows.

Despite the vastness of the African continent, Devil's Claw grows in relatively limited areas, and it is only found in Namibia (fomerly South West Africa), in the Savanna or Steppes of South Africa and the adjacent Kalahari Desert, in the south of Botswana and parts of the Transvaal and the north west region of the Orange Free State.

It belongs to a relatively small botanical family – the Pedaliaceae – and there are no known European representatives of this family. Like so many herbs, *Harpagophytum procumbens* has a number of names. Apart from the descriptive Devil's Claw it is also known as Wood Spider, Grapple Plant, Kalahari Skapkelu, Duiwelsdoring, Beestedoring, Kloudoring, Rankdoring, and, in German, Teufelskralle.

Although Devil's Claw was known to exist by botanists as long ago as the early nineteenth century, it was not until after the 1914-18 war that European attention was drawn to its medical properties. Such interest, at that time, was shown by G.H. Mehnert, a white farmer who had settled in what is now Namibia. Over a period of about forty years he studied the plant, the drying methods and the uses to which the natives put it, and he sent samples back to Germany for clinical trials. This was the next step towards the rightful recognition of the Devil's Claw plant, the first having perhaps been that fateful and unintentional one made by the primitive tribesman so very long ago.

The Vital Tubers

The long thin root of the Devil's Claw plant

gropes deeply down through the dry sandy soil to seek water and nutrients. At intervals side roots carry fleshy virile-looking white tubers which store food supplies for the prolonged droughts. These 'storehouse' tubers are the secondary roots and *it is only these tubers that contain the active and curative plant substances in usable amounts*.

In May of 1973 the results were published of examinations made by Dr Walter Shier and Hans Bauersfeld into two samples of *Harpagophytum procumbens*, both of which were being supplied for therapeutic use. They were concerned about the marked difference in appearance between the two samples. The first consisted of light-brown, fan-shaped pieces with curved surfaces – reminiscent of slices of mushroom, with an extremely bitter taste. On the other hand, the second sample was blackish-brown in colour on the outside and reddish-brown internally. The pieces took the form of long (2 in. or 6cm) slices of split root, and the taste was only faintly bitter.

After detailed examination – microscopically, chemically and chromatographically – they showed that, although both samples came from the Devil's Claw plant, the second less bitter specimen was from the main root and contained only small amounts of the active therapeutic constituents. The first sample, from the secondary tubers, was a powerful provider of the active ingredients.

Their conclusion was put in strong terms. 'Inclusion of the main roots must be looked upon as adulteration.' Fortunately, the taste and appearance of the true drug is distinctive and enables the very best makers of Devil's Claw products (such as Salus-Haus) to exercise stringent quality controls for the protection of the user. The tubers are first dug carefully from the soil and, after harvesting, they are thinly sliced and laid out to dry in the hot African sun.

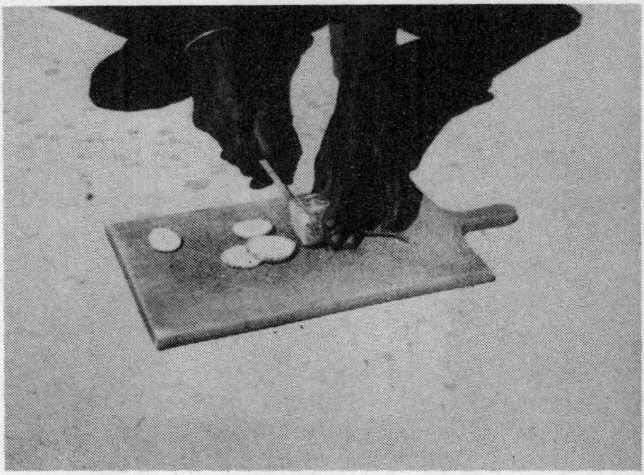

Slicing the secondary root of the Devil's Claw plant.

Fleshy Leaves

From the large bulbous root grow the young shoots, extending between one and one-and-a-half meters along the surface of the ground. The shoots are covered with fleshy leaves and attractive violet/red flowers, some four to six centimetres in length; looking rather like a bloom of a gloxinia or a foxglove. The woody fruits are between seven and twenty centimetres long, and carry four long spikes and many more that are two to ten centimetres long. They are very springy and extremely fiercely barbed. It is these fruits which damage so seriously the feet of man and beast.

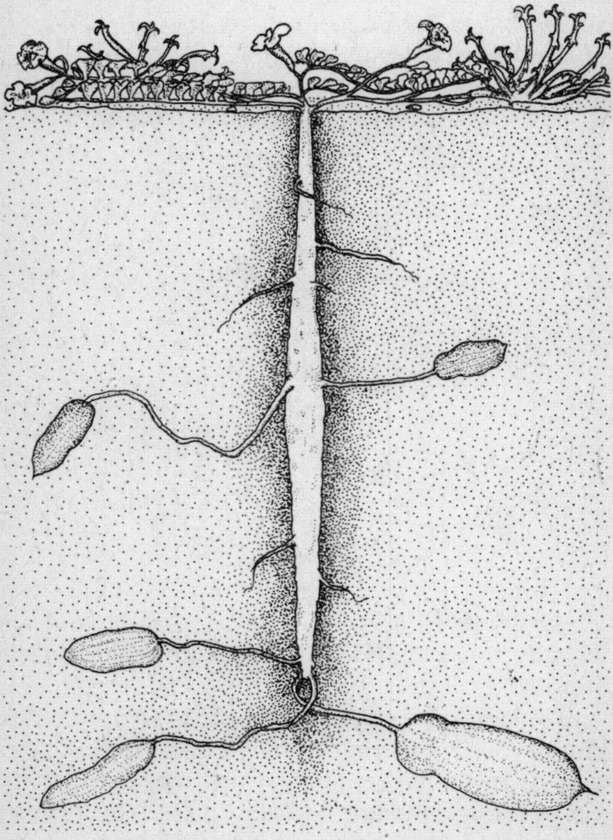

A Devil's Claw plant showing growth above and below ground.

The primary root goes down into the earth to a depth of between thirty centimetres and one-and-a-half metres, and at intervals secondary roots branch off bearing very large tubers which, when fresh, weigh as much as 600g ($1\frac{1}{2}$ lb). These tubers have a thin layer of cork round them to prevent them from becoming dry when, as is often the case, drought conditions persist for months at a time. The tubers range in colour from the lightest brown to a dark reddish brown. Should the protective layer become damaged, the high moisture content of the tuber makes it a good breeding ground for bacteria or fungi, and it is for this reason that, as soon as the tubers are lifted, they are sliced and sun dried.

The awful effects of the sharp claws on the feet of those who tread unwarily about the habitat of the Devil's Claw plant have already been described, but the worst economic problem associated with the plant today is the damage it can do to the feet of grazing sheep and cattle. Because of these dangers it can be foreseen that eventually particularly good growing areas will be fenced off and cultivated, but for the time being – certainly for the next few years – the plant grows wild and free like the animals of the jungle.

The genus *Harpagophytum* was first described in detail by von Burchell in 1822, and he called it by the name Uncaria, which came from the Latin *uncus* meaning a clasping hook. Sometime afterwards in 1845 de Candolle created the new name *Harpagophytum* which was a Greek translation of the English name for the plant at that time – the Grapple Plant.

The most modern review of this very small genus was undertaken by Drs Hans-Dieter Ihlenfeldt and Heidrun Hartmann of the University of Hamburg and it was published at the end of 1970. The authors examined virtually all the specimens available in all the herbaries of the world, as well as carrying out many studies in the field. They subjected the results of their work to modern statistical procedures and were able to show that there are, in fact, only two species of *Harpagophytum: procumbens* and *zeyheri*. These are divided into a further five sub-species and that is the full extent of the genus.

CHAPTER TWO
THE MEDICAL EVIDENCE

Since G.H. Mehnert first drew the attention of German pharmacologists to the remarkable results being achieved in Namibia with Devil's Claw, there have been a substantial number of medical trials – all of them so far successful. Work is still in progress, and there is more still to do – but there remains the fact that Devil's Claw is probably only exceeded by Ginseng in the amount of expert attention given to it during the past few years as a newly found or rediscovered natural remedy.

But why is it that so many medical discoveries seem to be national rather than international? As you will see later, the vast majority of the experimental work on Devil's Claw has been done in Germany. Luckily for us the Germans have a reputation for care and thoroughness. They are also well-known for their open-mindedness regarding the potential benefits of natural cures. I wonder if the same could be said of the majority of the medical and pharmaceutical experts in Britain and the United States?

Mehnert submitted those first samples, which he had been studying in Namibia for close on 40 years, to Professor Bernhard Zorn who is Director of the Physiological and Chemical Institute of the Friedrich Schiller University of

Jena. Professor Zorn was ready to make his preliminary communication to the professional magazine for rheumatic diseases on 9 September 1957.

Mehnert waited for the news with eager anticipation. Would the experience over hundreds of years by native sufferers be proved just another so-called placebo response where all that happens is that man is encouraged to mend himself? Or was Zorn going to find that Devil's Claw was indeed, as Mehnert thought, an important and significant step forward in therapeutics?

Zorn began his report by going over the story as it was told to him, saying that the plant was highly regarded by the African natives for its healing powers and was used as an infusion for rheumatic diseases, diabetes, arterio-sclerosis and diseases of the liver, kidneys and bladder. There were also, apparently, benefits to diseases of the stomach, the abdomen and the intestines. Claims were even made that the complaints of old age were improved by the regular use of the decoction. Hardened arteries became more elastic and there was a general feeling of well-being and strength.

Animal Trials

It was such reports as these, said Professor Zorn, that led his Department to carry out trials on animals. The tuber which he used had been prepared by Mehnert who had peeled, cut up, fermented and then dried it in the shade. Mehnert had told him that the method of use in

Africa was to infuse one to two heaped teaspoonsful of the resulting tea in a pint ($\frac{1}{2}$ litre) of boiling water in the evening, allowing the infusion to draw overnight. The resulting mixture is strained and then one third is drunk in the morning, one third at midday and one third in the evening.

To help test the anti-arthritic effects of the drug the technique used was to see if it relieved formaldehyde arthritis. This meant that the formaldehyde was injected into the heel joint of a rat causing an artificial inflamation and creating arthritis which reached its peak about a fortnight after the injection.

When the arthritis had reached its peak, treatment was begun; first of all by injection under the skin of ten arthritic rats. There were another ten arthritic rats which were not given the treatment so that they could be used as a control. He found that there was a pronounced reduction in the arthritic swelling as soon as the first injection was absorbed. With continued treatment the swelling reduced more and more and, even more surprisingly, when the treatment was discontinued the healing process continued.

After five weeks the swelling was only one-fifth as much as at the beginning and the rat's paws were fully mobile, while the untreated control-group rats improved hardly at all over the same period.

Professor Zorn next tried the administration of Devil's Claw by mouth. Here, except where the mixture upset the rats, results were almost as good, there being a one-third reduction in the swelling after only six doses by mouth.

He concluded that Devil's Claw contained a potent anti-inflammatory or anti-arthritic substance which could be extracted by infusion. He was especially interested in the fact that healing continued after the treatment was withdrawn and said that it was equivalent to the very best synthetic drugs in this effect. 'Lay opinions,' said Professor Zorn, 'concerning the healing properties of *Harpagophytum* root in rheumatic diseases can thus be accepted as true and are supported by our animal studies.'

Four years later Tunnman and Lux had isolated a possible active component called Harpagosid. Another two years passed by which time Lichti and Wartburg had worked out a formula for Harpagosid.

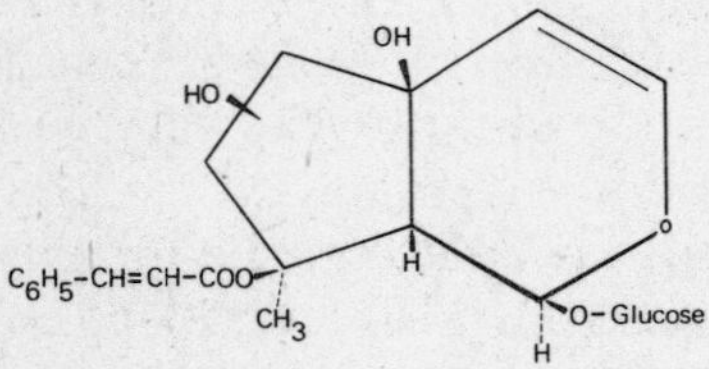

Structural formula for harpagosid.

A Renaissance of the Remedial Plant

The team of O. Eichler and C. Koch in 1970 tested the pure harpagosid to see whether the results established by Professor Zorn were also to be found in the pure substance that had been extracted from the Devil's Claw root.

First of all it was established that the toxicity

was low. In other words, Devil's Claw was a safe drug with which to experiment. They found that the results with pure harpagosid were very good but not nearly so good as when the whole extract was used: another example of the necessity for respecting the wholeness of nature.

At the same time they found that there was very little pain-killing effect from the herb, so the anti-arthritic results seen were not just as a result of the lessening of discomfort, but because of a real improvement in the condition. In that same year, 1970, Doctor Siegmund Schmidt published his results, 'A renaissance of the remedial plant!' He began: '*Harpagophytum* root provides us with an addition to our herbal armoury against the poisoning of modern times. It wonderfully stimulates the detoxicating and protective mechanisms of the body.'

This enthusiasm was not based on mere animal experiments. It came from day-to-day use by a famous medical practitioner and a leading expert in natural remedies.

Dr Schmidt had used a tea made from Devil's Claw for more than a year on over a hundred rheumatic patients. In some cases he has been able to entirely dispense with the use of other drugs, and in all cases found it to be a valuable support. Two years later Dr Schmidt wrote another paper confirming his earlier work and emphasizing how important it was that rheumatic diseases be brought under control because they were suffered by no less than 6 per cent of the world's population, about 150 million people! Indeed, in Germany where he was working they have one and a half million actually being treated for rheumatism and of these at least 10 per cent end up more or less immobilized.

He reported that Doctor J.R. Mose, who was Director of the Botanic Institute of Graz in Austria, had tested the root for its tolerance and found that even after long use there were no harmful effects. Dr Mose also found a slight cancer-inhibiting effect. But this is such a complex subject that I cannot deal with it in this short book.

God-Given Remedy

Dr P.C. Seeger prefaced his review in 1973 of *Harpagophytum an Effective Plant Remedy* with these words from the father of modern medicine, Paracelsus, who wrote 'God has not given us any disease for which he has not provided a remedy.' These words strike a resonant and responsive chord. Let us thank God that medical research is more and more turning to the proper use of the wonderful gifts of nature.

He said that the Benedictine expert on Tibetan and Indian medicine, Dr von Korvin-Krasinski, reported in a paper written in 1964 that Devil's Claw is a very good stimulant of the lymphatic system. This means that it helps the detoxicating system of the whole body. He went on to say that it brought about improvement in cases of disease of the gall bladder, pancreas, stomach and kidneys, and that avid users made infusions for diabetes, arterio-sclerosis, diseases of the liver, kidneys, bladder, stomach, intestines and abdomen as well as for the rheumatic conditions which are the principal use of Devil's Claw in the west.

Users must be warned, however, that diabetics should never take Devil's Claw except under strict medical control (for reasons explained on page 44). Dr Seeger went on to add up the results of Drs Amstein-Stauffacher (1961), K. Grunewald (1970), A. Beham (1971), W. Zimmerman (1971) and F. Schmidt (1972), all of whom reported excellent results when they used the herb in the treatment of rheumatic diseases, arthritis, arthrosis, diseases of the liver, gall bladder, stomach, intestines and kidneys in a total of more than 350 patients.

His own previous work had confirmed that many complaints of the liver, gall bladder and kidneys were relieved by Devil's Claw tea. He ascribed the beneficial effects of the herb to the chemical constituents which include harpagosid, harpagid and procumbin. There are other active substances which all contribute together, he believed, to the anti-arthritic and anti-rheumatic activity. This was partly because of the effect of an increased activity which Devil's Claw produces in the liver which detoxifies poisons such as urea, which is well known to have a part to play in rheumatic diseases.

It is so very interesting to see how, once again, the accurate observations of unsophisticated but wise people have been shown to be so right. A long tradition of herbal medicine produces not only safety but also effective healing action.

Dr Schmidt's Knee

It is entirely human that even the trained scientist becomes really enthusiastic about the treatment when it actually works on himself personally! A sudden shaft of the light of personal involvement illuminates the dry factual record of clinical cases.

Thus it was in the case of Dr F. Schmidt who treated 200 patients with rheumatic diseases over a period of three years by the use of Devil's Claw tea. He found that the tea had to be drunk for a sufficiently long time to be able to exert its influence and this depended on how severe the rheumatism was.

He recommended two to three teaspoonsful daily which were put with one litre ($1\frac{3}{4}$ pints) of boiling water and then left to stand overnight. The tea was drunk in small portions throughout the course of the day. The Devil's Claw tea did not only have an effect of its own, but also seemed to improve the results from using ordinary anti-rheumatic treatments so that freedom from pain and increased movement was obtained much more quickly.

He emphasizes that he did not believe that Devil's Claw alone could produce such rapid results, but he himself had pain on movement in his left knee which had not improved for two years and was particularly stiff in the morning. X-rays showed the early stage of arthritic change. Dr Schmidt had an injectable preparation of Devil's Claw prepared and injected 2ml on each side of the knee joint. After ten minutes the pain had gone and the knee was freely movable! Twenty-four hours later he repeated the treatment and this time the relief was extended to two days. He then increased the dose to 3ml either side and has now increased this to 6ml every three days. The knee joint is completely symptom-free, fully mobile and painless. Even more remarkable – the injections caused neither irritation nor pain.

Obviously any injections would have to be handled by a doctor, but as he found that the tea was also extremely effective this was a standard treatment for his patients.

Dr Schmidt also gave supporting treatment such as the use of special exercises, massages, hot baths, careful attention to diet and the addition of food supplements containing flower pollen. The detoxification of the patients was improved by a very nutritious diet which contained a lot of raw beetroot juice, yogurt-type foods and the use of plant oils such as sunflower seed oil together with the incorporation of as many raw foods as possible into the diet. He had found from experience that the use of pollen had a particularly good effect on the function of the liver so aiding the removal of poisons.

It is always important in the cases of rheumatic diseases of all types to try to restore the patient's weight to as near normal as possible because overweight throws unnecessary strain on the joints and muscles.

CHAPTER THREE

HOW SAFE IS DEVIL'S CLAW?

Almost everything we eat and drink is to some extent toxic. Our bodies can deal with certain quantities of all main food and medicinal substances without much trouble but there is a stage when even the most innocent ingredient becomes poison. For example a glass of whisky (if you like that sort of thing) can be a nice nightcap, but drinking a bottle of whisky is likely to spell disaster.

Potatoes contain the alkaloid solanine, and the amount of this substance is greatly increased if the potatoes are allowed to become green. Acute poisoning occurs from as little as 400 parts per million of the substance. Yet even fresh, good potatoes contain as much as 90 parts per million, so the margin of safety is not as great as you might imagine yet we all do eat and should eat potatoes with every enjoyment because of the very many good things that they contain – but do be careful that they are not green ones!

In the First World War the government recommended that people improve their diet by using rhubarb leaves as a green vegetable. This caused the death of several people and, as Dr Pyke reports, a woman in Montana died within 36 hours after eating a meal of fried rhubarb leaves. The stems contain lesser quantities of the toxic substance of oxalic acid but they, like spinach, should certainly not be fed to babies or to people who are short of calcium. Dr F.N. Strong in *The Journal of the Canadian Medical Association* showed that garden cress contained the poisonous substance benzyl cyanide in sufficiently large concentration so that one ounce could kill two mice.

In *The Journal of Human Nutrition* Professor Ian D. Morton, who is the Professor of Food Science at the University of London, gave a fascinating summary of some of these natural hazards to which we are exposed and, perhaps even more interesting, the way we have treated foods and drugs either by limiting the amount we take or by preparing them in some special way in order to make them relatively safe to live with.

We have all read of hippies going on 'trips' with LSD, but did you know that two average-sized whole nutmegs contain enough of a similar substance for most people to have hallucinations? In India a plant called the Chickling Vetch has been cultivated since ancient times as a valuable and useful protein supplement for a nation very dependent upon nutrition from cereals. This is all right when only a little is used in the diet, but in times of drought the plant grows very well and the poor people may eat more than half their diet from this one food. The result is a permanent muscular weakness and a paralysis of the lower leg. Yet another reason for keeping balanced quantities of many varied foods.

We are now eating more and more soya beans because this valuable food is not only very rich in high quality protein but also contains much very good unsaturated oil rich in linoleic acid, an important constituent of a good diet. It is not so widely known, however, that soya beans also contain certain toxic substances called lectins. These have the effect of preventing the efficient working of the natural human enzyme called trypsin which is essential to the digestion of protein. Happily these lectins are destroyed by moist heat, so remember to avoid raw soya beans!

No Side-effects from Devil's Claw

Now we must speak of Devil's Claw itself. Just where does this important medicinal plant lie in the scale of toxicity. Are we running into danger when we use it? The answer seems to be a resounding *no*.

Not one of the many medical research workers who have used Devil's Claw upon hundreds of patients has reported any untoward side-effects. Apart from the fact that it can only be given to diabetics under medical supervision, there are not yet any known reasons for not using Devil's Claw. This is in spite of the consumption of many millions of doses since the early 1960s.

These human experiences, however, are never enough nowadays to satisfy governments and officials. Animal experiments have to be done as well and indeed usually repeated in several countries and in several ways. One of the most important of these studies was carried out at the Laboratory for Pharmacology and Toxicology of Hamburg by Professor Dr F Leuschner who tested the toxicity of Devil's Claw in rats after giving it to them by mouth.

He gave three levels of dosage each to ten male and to ten female rats. The rats were starved for between fifteen and sixteen hours before the Devil's Claw was used, and this was administered by means of a tube so that the precise quantities needed for the experiment could be given with complete accuracy.

The rats were observed for four weeks when their general well-being, behaviour, food consumption and body weight were investigated. At the end of the experimental period the animals were dissected and closely examined. The lowest dosage given was 10,000mg per kilogram of body weight. The next was 12,600mg and the highest 15,900mg. This was the highest dose which Dr Leuschner could use because of the actual physical capacity of the rats. It is equivalent to no less than 1,272 grammes (or almost 45 ounces) in a fully grown man! Dr Leuschner concluded that none of these doses produced any symptoms of incompatibility. There were no adverse reactions of any sort and, although the quantities given were like multiplying the average daily dose in a human by some 1,500 times, there were no adverse findings.

CHAPTER FOUR

MANAGING YOUR ARTHRITIS

It is estimated that in the United States alone there are about 20 million sufferers from arthritis. This means that one in ten of the population suffers to some extent from arthritis and, of these sufferers, about fifteen out of every hundred are limited in their usual activity because of this disease. Women suffer more arthritis than men and 83 per cent of all cases are found in people who are more than forty-five years old.

The terms rheumatism and arthritis are used for many different diseases of the joints. Children and young people can suffer from rheumatic fever which has to be looked after very carefully indeed otherwise there is a danger that the heart will suffer. Fortunately, modern treatment has greatly reduced this threat.

Gout is another disease of the joints caused by a failure of the body's processes in the handling of uric acid. There are now a number of drugs which can help sufferers from gout, many made from natural materials. Devil's Claw has indeed been used for gout but so far no proper clinical tests have confirmed that it is really effective. This work still has to be done.

The most common type of arthritis is called osteoarthritis or, sometimes, degenerative arthritis. This is an arthritis typical of advancing years. It probably does not have any one cause but is a reaction against some of the stresses and strains experienced by most people as they become older. The apparent cause may be an actual injury or the pressure of over-weight or a bad posture; there may even be hereditary factors involved.

The first thing that happens is that the cartilage between the bones begins to degenerate. The joints that are commonly attacked are those of the fingers and thumb, and joints that carry the weight of the body such as the ankles, knees, hips and spine. First signs are often nothing more than a little stiffness when arising from a chair or after being in one position for some time. Later on there is soreness and inflammation which becomes less painful when the joint is in use and has been 'warmed up'. The condition is usually confined to the joints in which it first appears, and the use of Devil's Claw is certainly most helpful.

Because excess weight aggravates the condition, it is vitally important for the sufferer to try and reduce to a normal weight. In fact, it is sometimes found that this reduction brings about almost total relief from the pain. Here the reader must be warned against very rapid reduction through a crash diet. Such an attitude to slimming is usually doomed to long-term failure because it does not re-establish a normal eating pattern which is correct for the lifestyle of the person. A crash diet usually leads to an increase in weight when a normal eating pattern is resumed. It is much better to re-think your whole lifestyle and to reduce your weight very gradually by adopting a diet which is rich in whole, natural foods such as potatoes in their jackets, wholegrain bread, lightly cooked vegetables and salads, and plenty of fruit. Avoid useless fattening foods made from refined carbohydrates such as white sugar, white flour, strong alcoholic drinks and convenience foods where the convenience is to help the manufacturer rather than the nutrition of the consumer.

Rheumatoid Arthritis

Rheumatoid Arthritis is characterized by much inflammation and is often found in young adults, predominantly in women. The reason for it is not at all clear, although the idea has been put forward that it might be caused by a reaction of the body against certain of its own immune reactions or perhaps even because of an infection.

Sufferers often have to put up with tiredness, stiffness, pain – which may be considerable – and eventually deformity. This is especially obvious in the hands and knuckles which are often severely distorted and may become almost impossible to use. Normally, rheumatoid arthritis progresses unless treated, although the symptoms may disappear of their own accord for a while. The deformity cannot usually be cured because there are changes in the actual joints themselves. Nevertheless, Devil's Claw does help a large number of people to enjoy freer movement and a much easier life. It is important, as in the case of osteoarthritis, to reduce over-weight and to have an adequate and balanced healthy diet.

It is a good idea, if you are not a vegetarian, to have liver fairly often because this supplies valuable vitamin A, vitamin B complex and iron. Also arthritics are often known to be short of vitamin C so it is a good idea to take a natural vitamin and mineral supplement in order to make sure that there are no deficiencies.

It has been stated that almost half the people with rheumatoid arthritis overcome the disease because of the resistance of the body and a well-balanced diet supplemented with appropriate remedies. Sad to say there seems to be no very accurate way of deciding who will benefit from what treatment without trying it for yourself.

The Drug Treatment of Arthritis

As long ago as 1949 it was discovered that naturally occurring steroids such as cortisone were of considerable assistance in relieving the symptoms of rheumatoid arthritis. Such drugs often prevent the symptoms from developing or becoming worse, but when treatment is stopped the original disease often re-appears. Long-term treatment with cortisone and similar drugs often brings side-effects in its train. The bodily utilization of sodium and calcium can be affected and it is always wise when taking such preparations to avoid any added salt or the consumption of salt-containing foods. Some of the clinical tests with Devil's Claw have shown that it works well in patients who are taking cortisone and who are able thereby to reduce the amount they take thus limiting the possibility of side-effects.

Apart from cutting down on sodium it is also a good idea when taking this sort of drug, or indeed when taking aspirins, to make sure that they are only taken at the same time as a meal containing some protein such as fish, meat or cheese. Protein soothes the irritating effect of the drugs on the delicate linings of the stomach thus reducing the risk of tummy upset.

Food and the Kitchen

Many countries have voluntary agencies which run services such as 'meals on wheels', the purpose of which is to bring (often subsidized) food to those who are, through various incapacities, unable to prepare meals for themselves. It is very important that all old people and those of any age who are limited in their activities through arthritic diseases have at least one good balanced meal a day. Keeping food hot in order to get it to people's homes unquestionably causes certain losses in the vitamin and mineral contents so the previous advice given that you should take a vitamin and mineral supplement made from natural ingredients is wise, especially for the house-bound and elderly.

Your local public authorities will certainly have someone who is skilled in giving advice on the best way of preparing food and the best layout for your kitchen so that you can make the most of what movement you have. Very often quite small changes, such as the alteration in the height of drawers and tables and cooking facilities, or chairs made for easy mobility, can transform the amount you are able to do for yourself. If your hands are not very good it saves on the washing-up to prepare interesting one-dish meals such as casseroles.

If you do not meet many people and feel lonely do let voluntary aid organizations know about yourself. But above all try to retain interest in life and in the outside world. Many good cookery books take you round the world on a voyage of discovery. Do not be afraid to experiment with new dishes – there will, of course, be some disappointments – but you may find many that are evocative of half-remembered experiences with the pleasures and joys that they bring.

Devil's Claw Doses

Devil's Claw can be taken as a tea, in tablet form or by injection. As injections can only safely be given by qualified practitioners and because most tests have shown that to take Devil's Claw by mouth is quite as effective I shall not discuss the dosage of *Harpagophytum procumbens* by injection. As a matter of interest, for people who find that they have an uncomfortable reaction to taking Devil's Claw by mouth, it is possible to take it *per rectum*. This mode of administration is far more popular on the continent of Europe (for unfathomable reasons) than in either the United States or Britain.

I have mentioned in Chapter One that it is only the secondary roots or tubers of Devil's Claw that contain effective amounts of the active ingredients which help the arthritic sufferer. It is therefore very important only to use products which quite specifically state that they are made entirely from the secondary roots or tubers. If no statement to this effect is made on the packet, then beware in the absence of any evidence to prove the efficacy of the raw material.

The versions which I have seen made under extremely modern and laboratory controlled conditions are those produced by Dr Otto Greither at Salus Haus in Germany, and by Dr Dünner A.G. at Kirchberg in Switzerland. In both cases the batches of raw material are checked by the most modern means to ensure that they are up to the required standard.

Sad to say, random checks upon certain supplies of Devil's Claw available on the market show that some manufacturers do not have the equipment or do not take the care necessary to produce the high standard required for good results. It is always good advice to read the label before buying anything that you consume to make sure that the ingredients are good and safe and of the right sort and nowhere is this more important than with Devil's Claw.

Devil's Claw Tea

When taken in the form of tea made from tea-bags the average content of each bag is approximately 2½ grammes of dried secondary root. With this bag you make tea every evening before use. The filter bag is placed in a large glass or porcelain pot and to it is added ¾pt. (½ litre) of freshly boiled water. *The filter bag is left to infuse overnight.* The following morning the bag is removed and the resulting tea drunk in three equal portions (either cold or slightly warm) ten minutes before breakfast, lunch and the evening meal. Under no circumstances should the tea be boiled. Devil's Claw tea tastes exceedingly bitter but sugar has an adverse effect upon its qualities and so should not be added. The user will find that it is quite easy to become accustomed to this bitter taste and indeed many people eventually find it not unattractive.

Devil's Claw Tablets

The tablets are prepared by making an extract with water from the Devil's Claw tuber itself and, in fact, each tablet represents approximately 820 milligrammes of the active root, but this is concentrated to half that quantity. This means that one tablet contains just one third of the amount of active ingredient in a tea-bag. The tablets are taken in a similar way to the tea, that is to say that one tablet is swallowed with some liquid three times daily ten minutes before meals.

Duration of Course

The duration of the course of either the tea or the tablets is similar. Save in exceptional circumstances no real effects are observed for the first two or three weeks. But there is a build-up of the active principles in the body and usually relief follows. Most people find it best to go on taking Devil's Claw for nine weeks. There is no advantage whatsoever in increasing the dose above that which is recommended. At the end of nine weeks, your body will have built up a sufficient level of the active principles to allow you to discontinue taking Devil's Claw for two or three weeks.

This intermission between courses can be extended if you like, but most users find two or three weeks about right. The reason for the break is to avoid the chance of your body becoming accustomed to the effects of *Harpagophytum procumbens*. In other words you are giving yourself a slight rest and a chance to try to exist without the necessity for medicines. It is worthwhile reminding the reader that this is not a matter of safety, for Devil's Claw is one of the safest of the effective natural remedies.

Diabetics and Devil's Claw

Several times in this book the reader is warned not to take Devil's Claw if he or she is a diabetic. Diabetes is a disease in which the natural control of the level of sugar in the blood goes wrong. Many things affect this level, for example, a fever or a broken leg can alter the blood sugar level quite enough for a diabetic to have problems. The diabetes is controlled by the injection of insulin, the substance normally produced in the pacreas to control your blood sugar level, or through the use of tablets or simply by means of a careful diet in which the amount of sugars, and starches are accurately controlled.

The motto of the British Diabetic Association is 'balance is life'. The well-regulated diabetic has a good balance between his nutritional requirements, his insulin intake or tablets and his physical activity or state of health. Certain medical studies have shown that Devil's Claw can reduce the amount of insulin needed by the diabetic and is especially good in the case of diabetics who are also over-weight. Because the treatment of diabetes has to be a very accurate and highly controlled affair, I believe that it is not safe for diabetics to take Devil's Claw except under the most careful medical supervision. *Diabetics should definitely not take Devil's Claw for self-medication.* None the less if your doctor is interested and has the time and facilities to monitor your blood sugar level, then it may be possible that Devil's Claw will help both your rheumatic condition and your diabetes. This is another area in which more work is needed but the preliminary investigations are certainly most interesting.

CHAPTER FIVE

SOME BRITISH CASE HISTORIES

The clinical evidence from Germany was overwhelming. So fully was the folk medicine from Namibia supported by the experiences of highly qualified experts that news of the remarkable benefits to be gained from using Devil's Claw spread across Europe. The use of it was not just confined to natural practitioners but also the most orthodox doctors were convinced by the safety and reliability of this herb.

Tens of thousands had their sufferings relieved and many hundreds of these had been described in the medical literature as being greatly improved when normal medicines had previously had little effect.

Would the same story of success be repeated in Britain? It could be that the way people live is sufficiently different from that in Germany that the causes of the arthritis and rheumatism so effectively taken care of across the Channel were not to be repeated here. Because it was a newly introduced herb it was not permitted for advertising claims to be made for its effectiveness. British law is remarkably difficult when it comes to new medical developments, however safe they may be. But the product was made available both in tablet and in tea form. Some natural practitioners began to prescribe it for their patients and the good news began to spread by word of mouth up and down the country. There was no question but that here was another convincing step forward for natural medicine.

Statistics are vitally important but they lack human warmth. They are hard to relate to life. Orson Wells, playing the part of Harry Lime in the film *The Third Man*, gazed from the top of a fairground Big Wheel on the ant-like figures of the Viennese scuttling about far below, and posed the question that if one of those minute figures were to be 'snuffed out' who, from his high vantage point, would care? It is so hard to relate to hundreds of thousands of people dying of famine in some far off continent, and so easy when it is a beloved friend. Yet all life is important, as is all suffering. We must set out to relieve it where we can and how we can and it is much easier to do this when we can relate to actual experiences of people like ourselves.

So I have gathered together some case histories in the words of those who have used Devil's Claw. It is my hope that by passing on a few of these stories the advantages and indeed limitations of Devil's Claw will become more vividly recognized.

Arthritis

Mrs K.R. of Tralee.

> 'I have had very bad osteoarthritis and since I started *Harpagophytum* tea I have been able to stop taking drugs of every kind. I am really grateful for getting to know about *Harpagophytum*.'

Mr J.W. of Doncaster

'What wonderful results I have had from Devil's Claw tablets! I am 63 years old, and got laid up with arthritis, swollen-ankles, elbows and wrists. The Professor called it Poly-Arthritis. I could only walk about 100 yards and I had a lot of pain. Now I am almost back to normal! I do wish all arthritis sufferers would give them a trial. They would be so pleased with the results.'

Mrs E.F. of Cheshire

'We have used Devil's Claw tablets, for my husband's arthritis, he has now finished 28 days supply (84 tablets). We think that they are helping and though his legs are still bad the arthritis seems to have gone from his hands and the swellings have vanished.'

Mrs E. of Hyde

'I have now taken Devil's Claw tablets for six weeks with a week's break after three weeks. I have had great relief from arthritic pain, with considerable improvement of movement.'

Mrs J.A. of Bolton

'I have been taking Devil's Claw tablets for the last seven weeks and the pain from my arthritis is very much better. I would like to continue to take them permanently, so great has been the relief they have afforded.'

Mrs E.K.C. of Merthyr Tydfil

'I am on the last week of a nine weeks course of Devil's Claw for arthritis. My hands have improved considerably.'

Mr J.T. of Bristol

'I am suffering from Rheumatoid Arthritis and have been taking a course of Devil's Claw tablets. I am feeling much better, they do reduce the swelling of the joints. I had been suffering for some time.'

Mr A.T. of Liverpool

'I would like to take this opportunity to say that having completed a two month course of Devil's Claw tablets, there has been a great improvement in the Osteoarthritis in both my knees.'

Mrs P.S. of Eltham

'I have been taking Devil's Claw now for nine weeks, and have had some relief.'

Mrs E.V. of Bury

'I bought tablets of Devil's Claw at Bury Health Food Stores. I began treatment on December 3rd 1976 for Arthritis of the top of my shoulders and after one week the pain had gone.'

Mrs G.K. of Broseley

'I have been taking drugs from the doctor for years, am crippled with arthritis and I cannot go out. I was told about the Devil's Claw. So I was able to get 84 tablets and am now nearly to the end of same. I have not taken any drugs since I started Devil's Claw and I do feel much better and more free from pain.'

Mr R.S. of Rayleigh

'I have had Rheumatoid Arthritis for over 15 years I have had all kinds of treatment but with no improvement. I heard about Devil's Claw for arthritis. I have taken these pills for the course of nine weeks. I have had a lot of improvement.'

Mrs W.J. of Caernarvon

'My thumb is so painful that my writing is bad but I'm glad to say it has improved since taking the Devil's Claw tea.'

Mr A.B. of Huddersfield

'My wife suffers from arthritis, mainly in the hip and has completed an eight week course of the tablets which, I am pleased to say, has given some relief.'

Mrs M.B. of Wilmslow

'I have suffered from arthritis for a few years. Having bought Devil's Claw I am now getting much less pain.'

Mrs T. of Hampshire

'I feel very strongly that this root should be televised or somehow brought to everyone's knowledge, especially the doctors and surgeons of this country. The people that I know who live alone, who have been suffering terribly distressing diseases and having to go through terrible operations, having their insides replaced, and more or less turning people into guinea pigs. The suffering experienced through these operations can't be described, and I am sure could be done without if this root was taken instead.

'My mother has had four weeks treatment of the Claw, i.e. three tablets per day, one taken ten minutes before meals, and is going to reduce the dose to two per day for four more weeks. She is then going to stop taking them. We and she just can't believe the difference: four weeks ago she was laying for two weeks speechless and exhausted, and going mad with the terrible burning intense pain all over her head, arms, body and legs, and with the pain and awful tingling her nerves were broken. We couldn't leave her bedside as she also felt as if her chest was closing in, and the intense pain in her chest was almost suffocating her, she just hadn't the strength to breath, and it was heartbreaking to watch her, having been in this state for three months. She has had a crumbling spine for 30 years, and now the vertebrae which hold the balance of the whole body have disintegrated, causing the bones to press on the nerves, which are now exposed, therefore causing inflammation and pain and shaking (the arthritis had set in all up her spine where it was decayed) and was all over her body. This has all stopped and disappeared. She is running about like a ten year old. She is keeping a box handy in case any more pain comes (which it could because of her bone condition). I just can't find words to describe this wonderful miracle. Her sight has improved, and she felt hungry after two weeks treatment, which she hasn't done for years: she has only eaten a child's meal really, having always felt so sick with pain. Now she is cake-making and cooking meals, and looking after herself more.

Another case of a woman with the same complaint, but in an earlier stage – she could not lift her arms and was in constant pain from her back, and dragging swollen legs. I told her what I was giving mother (whom she saw when very ill and thought she wasn't going to live much longer, and saw her two weeks later after two weeks of treatment, up and about, bright and lively.) She started taking the claw and after taking only five tablets could lift her arms very easily and her legs and was free of pain, in fact she came dancing in the door like a child; she was so excited, she has, like me, told everyone she can get hold of on her travels.'

Gout

Mr G.T. of Manchester

'I have been taking Devil's Claw for nearly nine weeks and although it has not cured my condition, which is gout, I am very much improved.'

Psoriasis

Mrs M.L. of Bury

'I suffer with psoriasis. After taking the tablets for three weeks there is a great improvement.'

Rheumatism

Mr S.G. of Notthingham

'I have suffered with rheumatism in both my upper arms and shoulders for the past eight years, which I believe originally started by being in a car whilst the windows were open. I tried everything to cure this but to no avail and when I consulted my doctor about this recently he said nothing could be done and all he was able to do was give pain killers. I started taking Devil's Claw tablets in November last year and after some six weeks noticed that the twinges were getting less and less severe until I very rarely suffered at all. I stopped taking the tablets and after a couple of weeks I noticed a slight return of the rheumatism in my right arm, I restarted the tablets and the pains again disappeared.'

Mrs D. of Repton

'I have had a very hard year with rheumatism. I was advised to try Devil's Claw tea, the result is that I am moving much more freely.'

Poor Circulation

Mrs M.T. of Chorley

'I sent to Switzerland for the herb which I received after much trouble. I took the herb as per instructions and after three weeks break as told to do, I carried on taking it. I have found it very beneficial generally. My problem was poor circulation and I know I have been better since taking *Harpago*.'

Back Sores

Mr E.R. of Torquay

'I have made a paste of Devil's Claw tablets each day and put it on the two sores on my back which I have had for a long time and am able to report that they really do look better and feel better.'

Nervous Stomach and Poor Digestion

Mrs J.W. of Abergele

'My husband and I decided to try Devil's Claw and we were both impressed by how it worked even after the first box (15 sachets). We are now on the second box and although I find it bitter to take, I mean to stay the course. We find it very good for digestion and it seems to stop the nervous stomach as well as making us feel good generally.'

General Health

Mrs J.C. of Maidenhead

'I have been taking Devil's Claw Tea for three weeks and am happy to say that my general health is much improved.'

These are just a small selection of the very many reports I have from those who have successfully used Devil's Claw. You will notice, and this is not surprising considering the wide variety of uses, that some have only experienced a little improvement whilst others have results which can only be called spectacular.

Of course when the popular press finds a well-known sportsman who recovers from being crippled with arthritis and is able to play again, they make the most of it! League footballer George Sutherland from Inverness hit the headlines during September 1977. Here are some typical news items which speak for themselves – and for Devil's Claw!

An Inverness newspaper said:

GARLIC AND DEVIL'S CLAW
GET NORTH MAN BACK ON HIS FEET

Inverness Welfare League footballer, George Sutherland, once a martyr to arthritis believes he may have found a 'horror cure' – garlic, a well-known protection against vampires, and Devil's Claw tablets. Three years ago Mr Sutherland was struck with arthritic pains in his shoulder, back, ankles and feet. The pain was so bad that he thought he would have to give up work. Special drugs recommended by doctors, heat treatment and even special diets of brown rice and fish were all tried by Mr Sutherland, purchasing manager at an Inverness hotel. Still the pain became worse. But later this month George will put on his football boots and take to the field.

'Six months ago it was agony to stand on my feet, but now I can jump the garden fence with ease,' said George of 32 Drynie Avenue, Inverness. The secret of his amazing 'cure', George thinks, is based on two herbs which can be bought at any health food store. After five months on these tablets the pain vanished. 'It was extremely sudden," he said. 'One morning I woke up and, while there was still pain, the agonising sharpness was gone. I am convinced this herbal recipe could help others.'

'I would say this was a cure and not just a pain killer. But if bones are bent by the disease the herbs will not straighten them. If it is caught early on I think it could help other sufferers.' George takes three garlic tablets before going to bed and three of the Devil's Claw during the day. 'They must stick to the course of tablets,' he said, 'It was five months before they worked with me.'

Dr W.M. Lancaster of Inverness Royal Northern Infirmary, who treats many rheumatic and arthritic patients, said this morning that offhand he could not say if this was a cure or not.

'But it is working for Mr Sutherland, by all means he should continue with the tablets', he said. 'I would really like to know more about this case.'

A further report in the paper said:

THOUSANDS WANT CURE

An Inverness Welfare League footballer's amazing cure from arthritis has raised the hopes of sufferers throughout Scotland. Mr George Sutherland (36) 32 Drynie Avenue, Inverness, has received 4,500 letters from people seeking his cure which is based on two herbs – garlic and Devil's Claw. 'The response has been fantastic, it shows the many people who are desperate to be cured. I know the pain these people are experiencing as I suffered for three years.' He and his family only recently moved house and their home improvements are being temporarily delayed until the letters are answered. The hallway is a sea of unopened letters and a ground-floor bedroom is also being used as a store. To ease the problem of answering the letters Mr Allan Sellar the proprietor of the health food shop where Mr Sutherland bought his ingredients has reproduced 2,500 copies of Mr Sutherland's letter detailing the cure.

Mr Sutherland assisted by his wife and four friends, began answering the mail on Monday night. 'We were working until after midnight and managed to answer 500 letters.'

Mr Sutherland is convinced the herbs will help those plagued with arthritis. He took three Devil's Claw tablets and three garlic oil capsules each day for five months, laying off fizzy drinks. He began the medication after all other treatment failed. One day he woke up and the pain was gone. Mr Sutherland plays his first game of football next Wednesday.

Another newspaper reported:

GEORGE IS BACK ON THE BALL...
and he puts it down to Garlic
and Devil's Claw

Three years ago Welfare League footballer, George Sutherland, was struck with Arthritis, causing him severe pain in his shoulder, back, ankles and feet. The pain was so bad that George thought he would have to give up work. Special drugs recommended by doctors, heat treatment and even special diets of brown rice and fish were all tried by Mr Sutherland. Still the pain became worse.

But later this month, George will put on his football boots and take to the field, and he has already been out for a practise jog.

'Six months ago it was agony to stand on my feet, but now I can jump the garden fence with ease.' said George.

It was through experimenting with various herbs, some recommended by Barbara Cartland the health food expert, that George discovered garlic and the claw tablets was his cure.

World Famous Chef's Discovery

The millions of readers of *The Daily Express* of London saw on 10 December 1977 an article by Adella Lithman saying how Monsieur Jean Conil brought the crippling rheumatism of his Irish wife Mary under control with Devil's Claw and a reformed diet.

He describes how his wife had suffered for years, and, in spite of great efforts the doctors had not been able to do very much to help. He thus started to look for alternatives and gave the whole subject of rheumatic diseases much thought. Dwelling on the argument that most rheumatic and arthritic conditions are precipitated by stressful conditions, by wrong eating habits and through a general mismanagement of life itself, his mind went back to his old grandmother who made tisanes of herbs lovingly grown in her own market garden in France. His belief in a sympathetic understanding of nature and its wonders eventually led him to try out Devil's Claw.

The results were dramatic in that his wife's condition improved within a few short weeks. An improvement that has since been maintained.

But that was not enough. Monsieur Conil understood that the simplest and most effective cure must be to reform the diet. To have an improved diet *and* Devil's Claw – that could be an even better answer.

He spoke of the years of pain his wife had suffered and of the thousands of pain killing tablets which she had to take to make life bearable. Monsieur Conil himself uses the traditional remedy of a week eating nothing but grapes when he himself feels ill and, although he was emphatic in pointing out that his ideas could not cure distorted limbs nor remedy disfigured joints, he had tried out the combined Devil's Claw and diet therapy on about a hundred of his friends and in most cases the results had been very good.

Whilst he enjoys meat, he believes that rheumatic sufferers should eat less meat and more fish and vegetables. He is also very keen on the new soya protein foods, especially when they are flavoured naturally. Indeed, Jean Conil is sure that we must get back to more natural food and avoid the refined and sophisticated convenience products on today's supermarket shelves.

The foundation of his dietary support to Devil's Claw is 'The Conil Miraculous Salad,' the ingredients of which are:

Watercress
Lettuce
Raw Spinach
1 sliced Avocado
2 sliced Tomatoes
½ small Cucumber (sliced)
4 oz. (100g) sliced Celery
1 sliced Apple (with skin)
1 medium-sized Onion (sliced)
5 oz. (150g) sliced Pineapple (must be fresh)

Dressing:
¼ oz. (6g) fresh Ginger
1 clove of Garlic
1 oz. (25g) chopped Onion
4 oz. (100g) fresh Pineapple (diced)
5 fl.oz. (150ml) fresh Pineapple Juice
Juice of a Lemon
2 tablespoonsful Salad Oil
5 fl.oz. (150ml) plain Yogurt
Salt and Pepper to taste

Mix all the main ingredients together. Be sure they are well sliced, and put them into a salad bowl. Liquidize the dressing mixture, and pour into the bowl. Toss the salad and dressing together and serve, decorated with sliced hard-boiled eggs and toasted peanuts. He suggests that such a salad be eaten once a day.

Monsieur Conil has many gold medals which bear witness to his culinary expertise – but my belief is that in the future his true memorial will be seen in the many things he has done and is doing to help sufferers from rheumatic diseases. He has already launched a research fund to help buy a £100,000 scanning machine for a London Hospital.

He says that he has found that two or three tablets of Devil's Claw a day, or one pint of Devil's Claw tea seems about right. After nine or ten weeks he recommends that people leave off the Devil's Claw treatment but keep on with the diet for two or three weeks, and then go back to more Devil's Claw.

It is remarkable that Monsieur Jean Conil, the great, great, great, great grandson of Louis Conil, chef to Marie Antoinette and Louis XVI, found intuitively the same methods of administration that the research workers in Germany had spent so much time arriving at through clinical experimentation.

SELECT BIBLIOGRAPHY

Abou-Mandour, A. 'Pharmazeutisch-Biologische Untersuchungen der Gattung *Harpagophytum*' (Tissue cultures of H.p.), *Planta Medica,* Vol. 31, pp. 238-244 (1977)

Czygan, F.C., and Krüger, A. 'Distribution of the glycoside Harpagosid in the different organs of H.p.', *Planta Medica,* Vol. 31, pp. 305-307 (1977)

Dittrich, C., '*Harpagophytum procumbens* D.C.', *OAZ,* p. 54

Editorial, 'Sie sind keine placebos', *Euromed,* No. 15, pp. 631-632

Eichler, O., and Koch, C., 'Uber die antiphlogistische, analgetische und spasmolytische Wirksamkeit von Harpagosid', *Arsneim-Forsch (Drug Res.),* Vol. 20, No. 1, pp. 107-109 (1970)

Hager, *Handbuch der pharmazeutischen Praxis,* 9th edn., Vol. 5, pp. 18-20, Springer Verlag 1976

Hoppe, H., *Einfluss der Droge Harpagophytum procumbens D.C. auf Diabetes Mellitus mit Fettstoffwechselstörungen, Erfahrungsheilkunde,* pp. 230-233 (1974/7)

Ihlenfeldt, H.-D., and Hartmann, H., 'Die Gattung *Harpagophytum* (Burch.) D.C.' *Meissn. Mitt. Staatinst. Allg. Bot. Hamburg,* Vol. 13, pp. 15-69 (1970)

Korvin-Krasinksi, P.G., *Tibetanishe Medizinphilosophie II,* Origo Verlag, Zurich (1964)

Leuschner, F., *Akute Toxizitat von 'Teufelskralle' an Ratten bei Peroraler Verabreichung,* private communication

Schier, W., and Bauersfeld, H., 'Handelsorten von

Harpagophytum procumbens D.C.', *Deutscher Apotheker-Zeitung,* No. 21, pp. 795-796 (1973) and No. 45, pp. 1800-1801 (1974)

Schmidt, S., 'Phytotherapie beim rheumatischen Formankreis', *Erfahrungsheilkunde,* Vol. 5, pp. 152-154 (1973/5)

—*Rheumatherapie mit Harpagophytum Therapiewoche,* Vol. 72, pp. 1072-1074 (1972)
Therapiewoche, Vol. 72, pp. 1072-1074 (1972)

Schroedter, A., 'Zur Atiologie, Diagnostik und Therapie der progredient chronischen Polyarthritis', *Volksheilkunde,* Vol. 26, No. 3, pp. 66-105 (1975)

Seeger, P.G., '*Harpagophytum,* ein wirksames Phytotherapeutikum', *Erfahrungsheilkunde,* Vol. 8 (1973)

Sticher, O., 'Die aktuelle Droge: *Harpagophytum procumbens', Deutscher Apotheker-Zeitung,* No. 32, pp. 1279-1284 (1977)

Tunman, P., and Hammer, H.-E., 'Konstitution des Procumbids', *Liebigs Ann. Chem.,* Vol. 712, pp. 138-145 (1968)

— and Lux, R., 'Zur Kenntnis der Inhaltstoffe aus der Wurzel von H.p. D.C.', *Deutscher Apotheker-Zeitung, pp. 1274-1275 (1962) and pp. 395-397 (1963)*

—and Stierstorfer, N., 'Uber ein weiteres Glukosid', *Tetrahedron Letters,* No. 25, pp. 1697-1699, Pergamon Press

Vogel, A., '*Harpago,* Teufelskralle', *Kurier,* No. 113 (1973)

— 'Teufelskralle-Tee', *Gesundheits-Nachrichten,* Vol. 7 (1973)

Volk, O.H., 'Zur kenntnis von *Harpagophytum procumbens* D.C.', *Deutscher Apotheker-Zeitung,* Vol. 18, pp. 573-576 (1964)

Watt, J.M., and Breyer-Brandwijk, M.G., *Medicinal and Poisonous Plants of Southern and East*

Africa, p. 830, Edinburgh, London, 1962

Zimmerman, W., 'Erfahrungen mit *Harpagophytum*', *Physikalische Medizin und Rehabilitation*, Vol. 7, pp. 317-319 (1977)

Zorn, B., 'Uber die antiarthritische Wirkung der *Harpagophytum*-Wurzel', *Zeitschrift fur Rheumaforschung*, Vol. 17, pp. 134-138 (1958)

N.B. Most of the original papers on Devil's Claw are written in German, and should any reader seek further information the above is a comprehensive list. All of these sources have been referred to in the course of writing this book, and in addition more than thirty other papers were researched.

INDEX